Co

©2019, Miranda Watson and James Rosone, in conjunction with Front Line Publishing, Inc. Except as provided by the Copyright Act, no part of this publication may be reproduced, stored in a retrieval system or transmitted in any form or by any means without the prior written permission of the publisher.

ISBN: 978-1-957634-28-9
Sun City Center, Florida, USA
Library of Congress Control Number: 2022904128

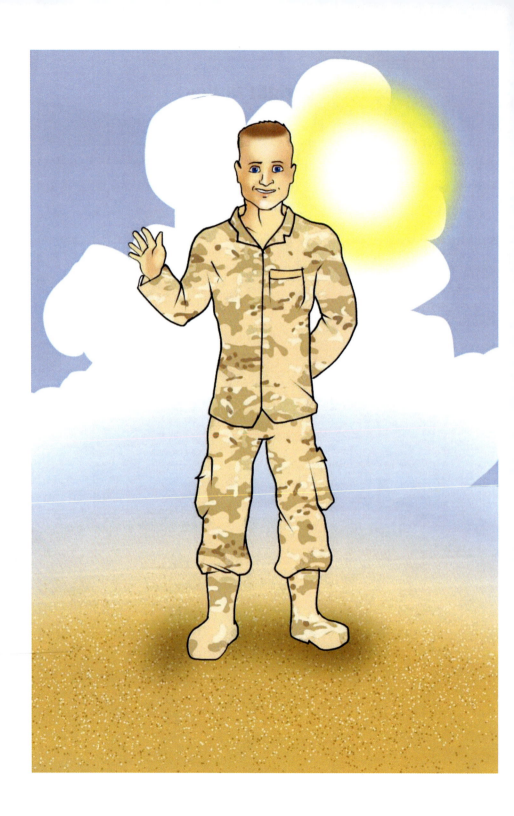

My Daddy works as a soldier for the United States military.

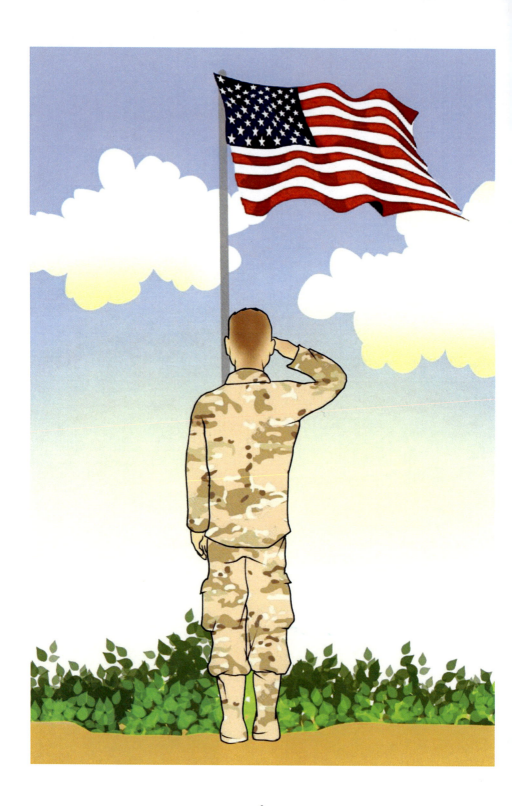

He is proud to serve our country and to protect our freedoms.

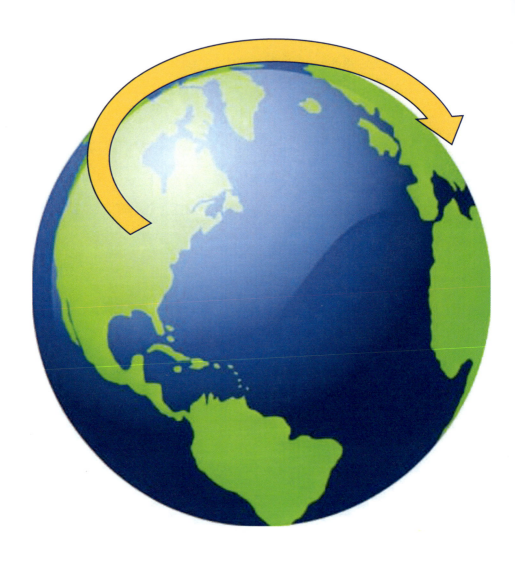

Daddy went to Iraq as part of his job. Iraq is very far away, and he was gone for a long time.

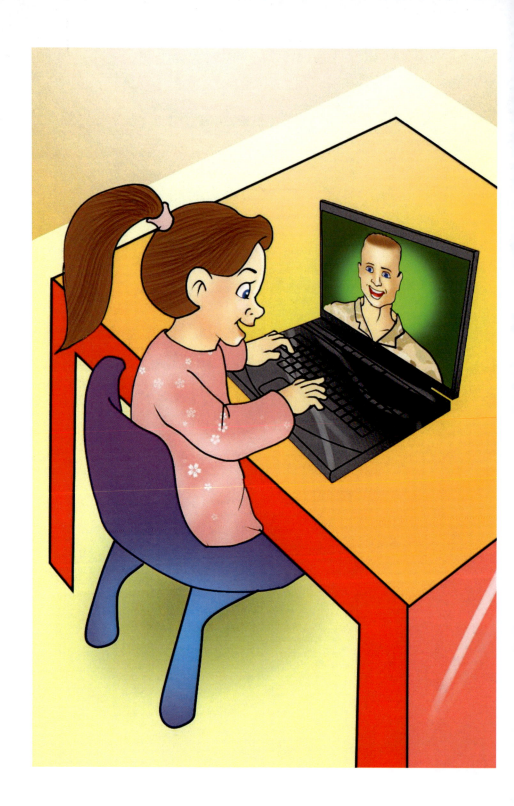

I missed my Daddy very much. We would talk on Skype sometimes, but I still wanted him to be home.

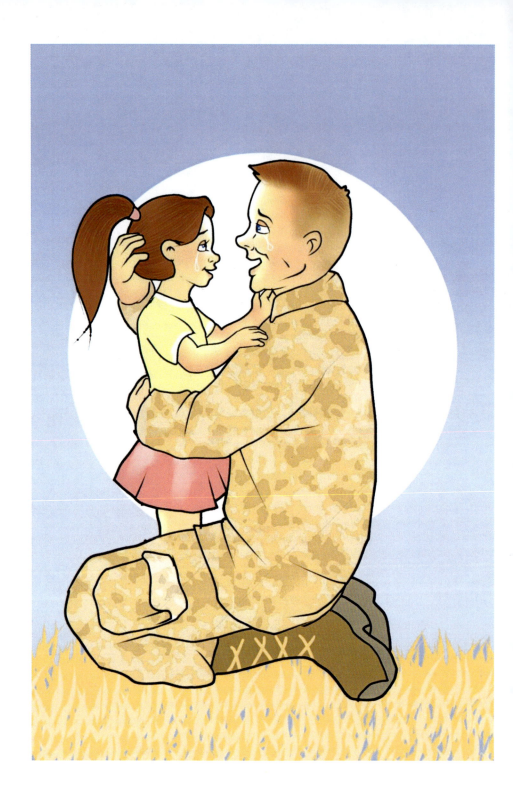

Daddy was finally done with his job there and flew back to America. I was so happy to see him and hug him in person! And he was happy to see me too.

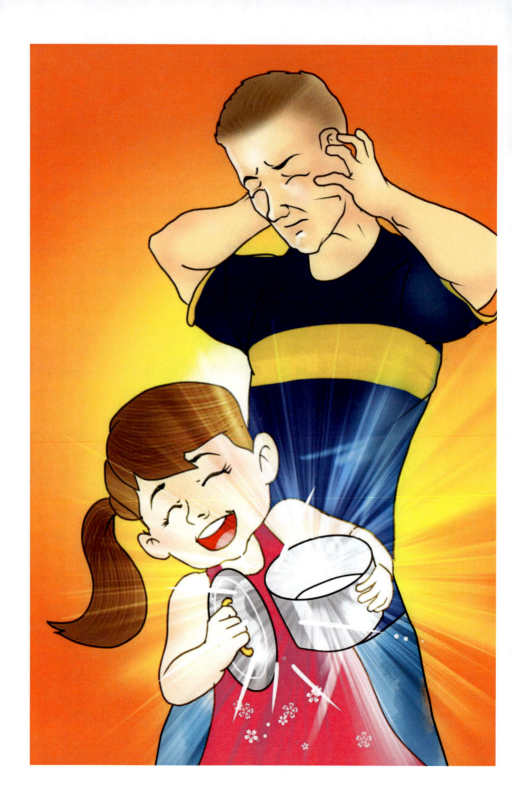

But Daddy was different when he came home. He got angry a lot more easily than he used to. One day, I made a loud noise while playing and he yelled at me. That made me feel sad and afraid.

Daddy never used to yell at me when I made loud noises before.

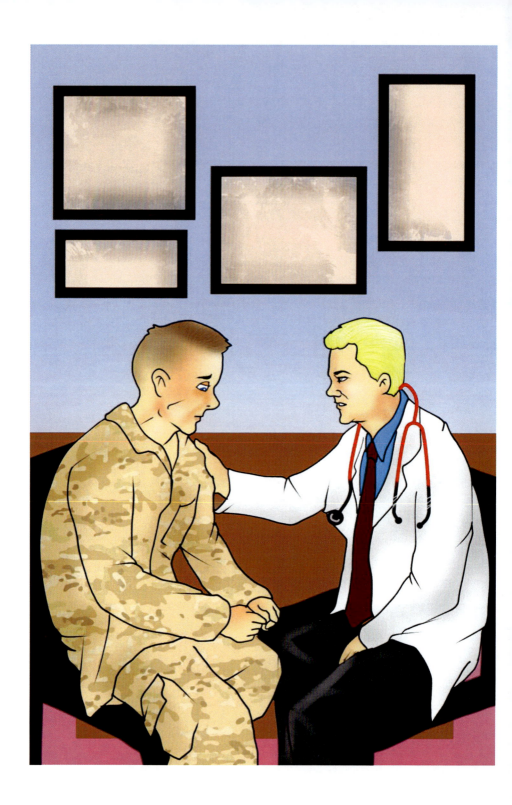

Daddy realized that he needed some help and started seeing a doctor that helps with your mind. The doctor explained to my Dad that he has PTSD or post-traumatic stress disorder.

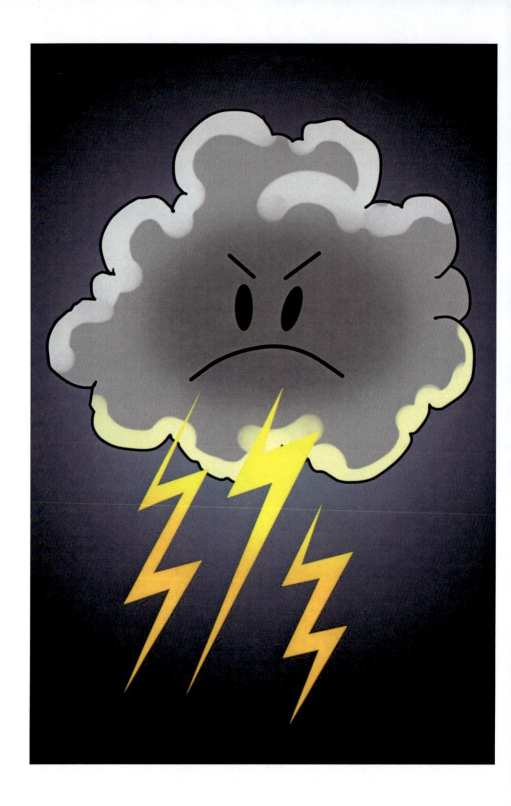

Some very horrible things happened to my Dad while he was away—things that he doesn't want to talk to me about. He doesn't want to make me feel frightened, but he does talk to his special doctor about what happened.

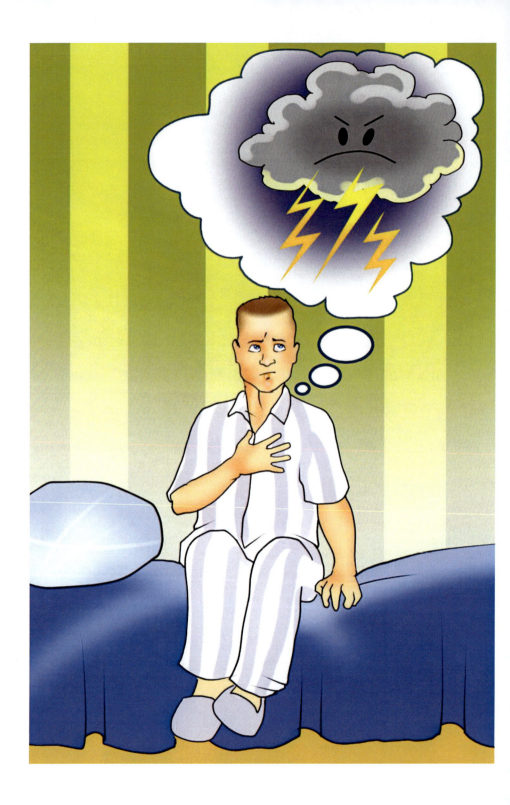

He keeps having bad dreams about what happened, and sometimes things going on around him trigger a bad memory. When that happens, he feels like he is in danger. He feels like someone might hurt him. He feels like the bad memory is happening again.

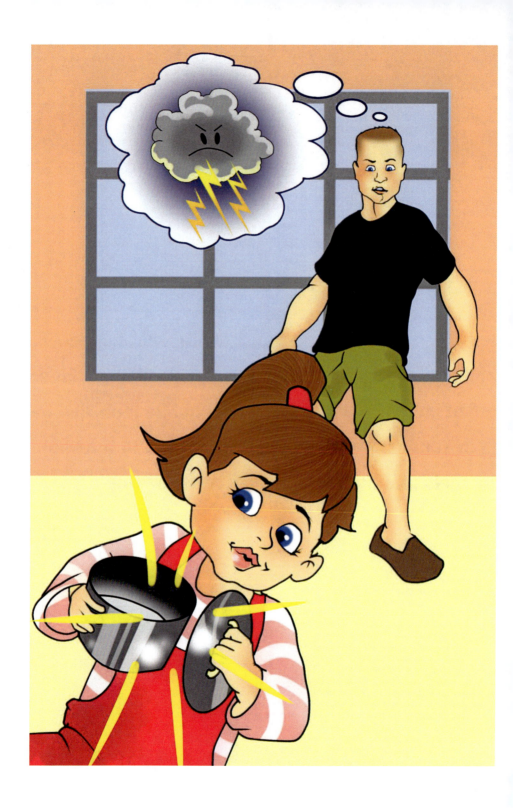

When I made a loud noise, my Daddy's mind went back to the bad memory. It wasn't my fault that this happened to him, but he will need help to make it stop.

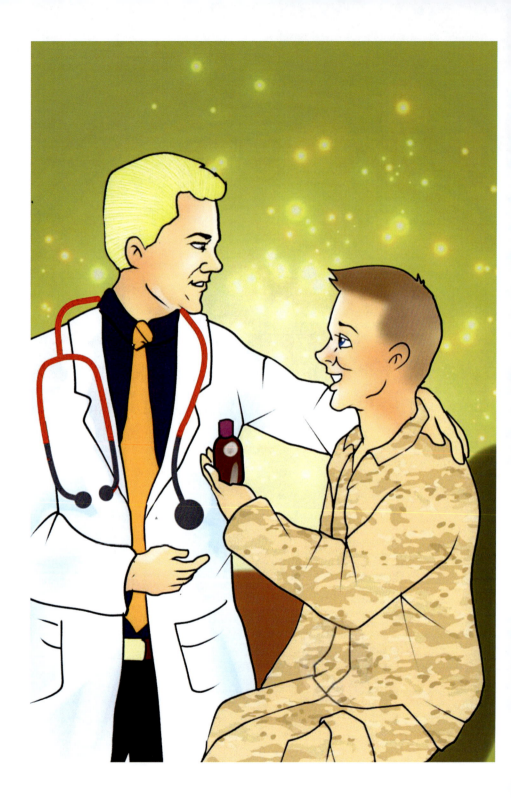

The special doctor told my Dad that there are a lot of ways that he can start to feel better, and he is working hard to make that happen. He sees a counselor and takes special medicine now that helps him to be calmer.

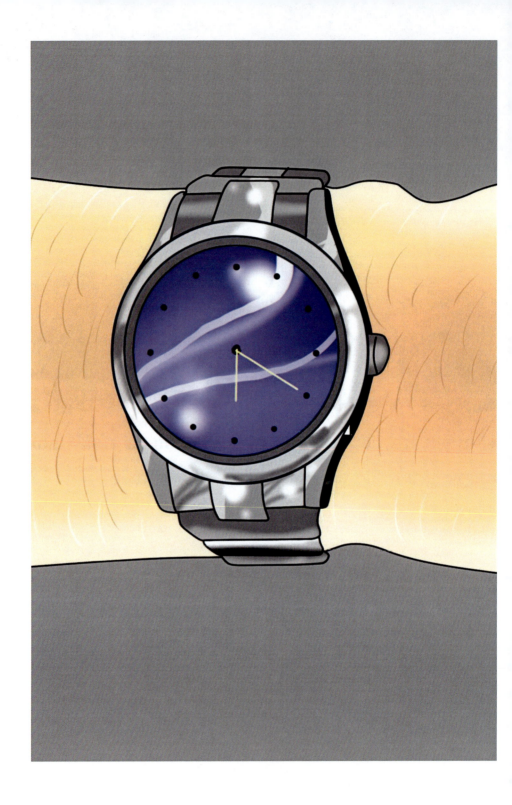

One thing he learned is that sometimes, when there is a loud noise or some other trigger that starts the bad memories, he will need to take some time to calm down.

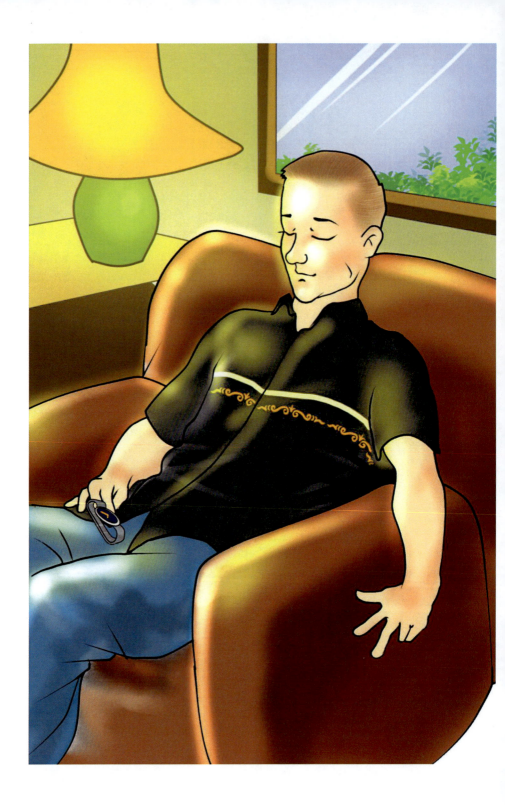

Sometimes my Daddy goes to the other room and does some deep breathing exercises. He might close his eyes and count. Sometimes he prays.

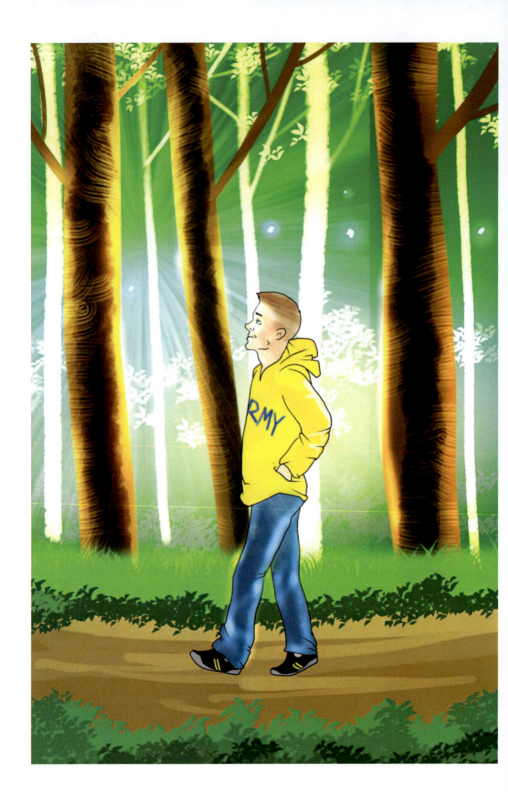

Sometimes Daddy goes for a walk by himself to calm down.

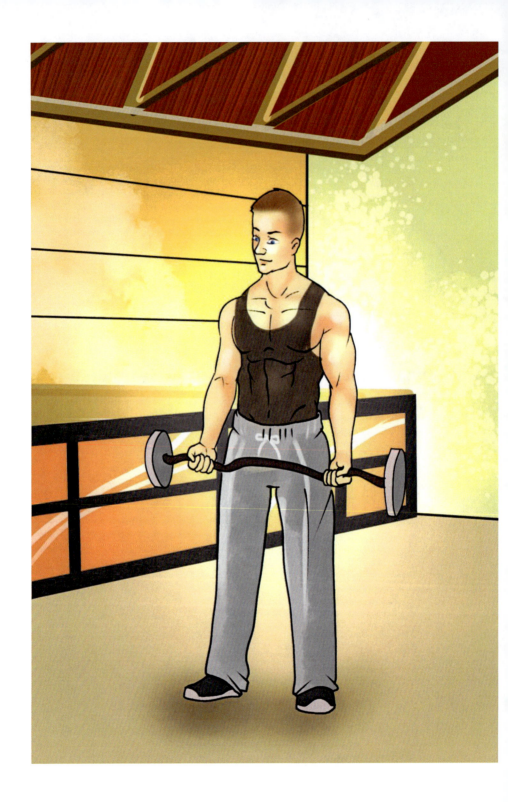

Sometimes Daddy works out in the garage for a little while.

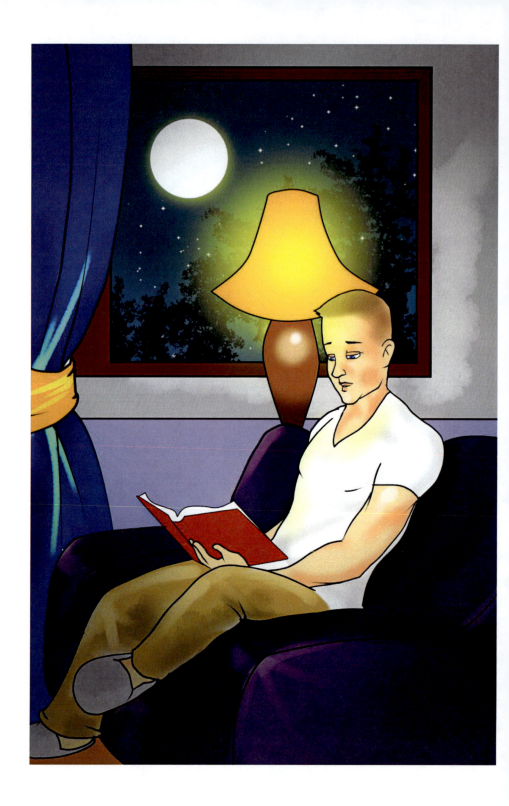

Sometimes he reads a book or plays a video game until he feels calm again.

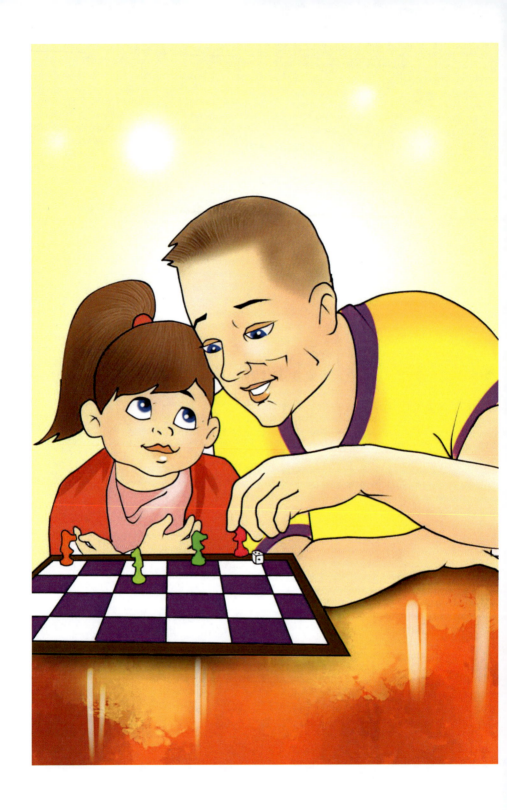

When his body and mind have calmed down, then he can come back and play with me again. My Daddy still loves me and wants to spend time with me.

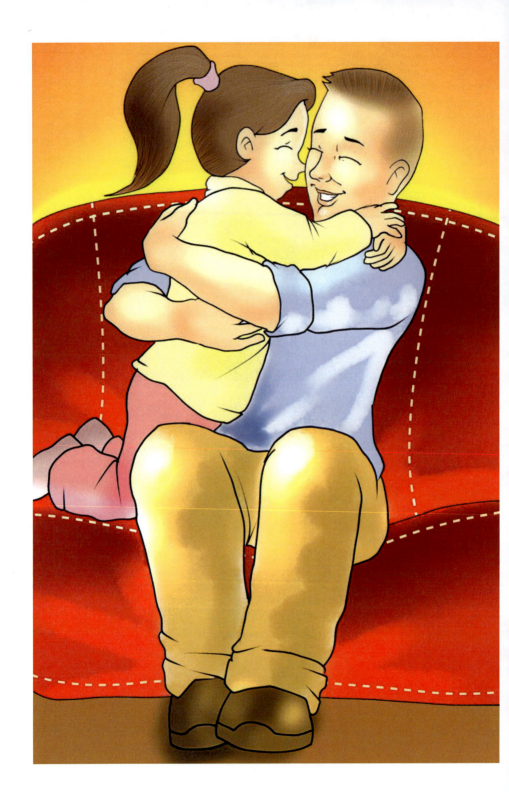

I know my Daddy is not the same, but he is working hard to be the best Daddy he can be. He still gives me hugs and lets me know he loves me, and I can tell him how I feel too.

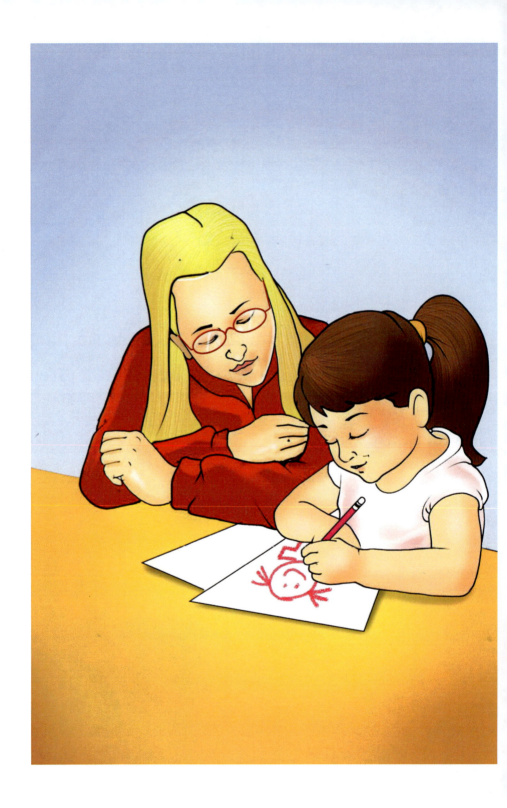

I needed some help to understand what was happening with my Daddy, so I went to go talk to a special doctor too. That's OK. It's good to get help when we need it.

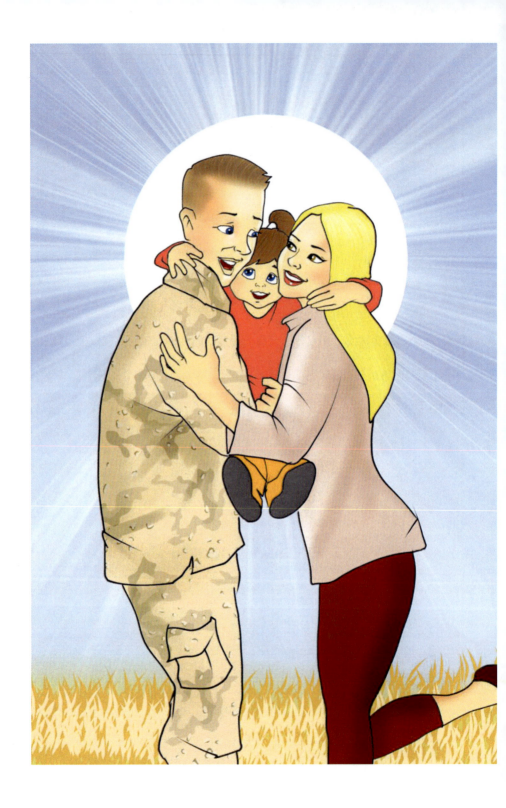

I love my Daddy, and my Daddy loves me. Things may be different now, but that's OK. We are learning how to move forward as a family.

Conversation Starters

1. What is one thing you like to do to help yourself calm down?

2. Can you think of one new way you could try to help your body feel calmer?

3. What is one new way you could help calm your thoughts?

4. How does your Mommy or Daddy calm down?

5. What is one way you can build a positive memory with your Mommy or Daddy?

A Place to Draw or Write your Feelings

For the Adult:

Post-traumatic stress disorder can cause a variety of symptoms, including recurring nightmares of traumatic events, insomnia, hypervigilance, flashbacks, depression, agitation, irritability, and anxiety. For some, these "fight or flight" responses occur very frequently and can impact every aspect of that person's life.

Fortunately, there is help. If you, or someone you love, is dealing with PTSD, here are some options:

1. The VA offers the following types of help: medication management, talk therapy, cognitive processing therapy or CPT (usually done in a group setting), prolonged exposure therapy, anger management group sessions, and PTSD symptom management group sessions. These services are available to all veterans at no cost.

2. The Vet Center is paid for by the VA but is not attached to the VA hospital. A veteran can use their benefits for free as long as they produce a DD214. Some of the therapies they provide include: CPT group sessions, eye movement desensitization and reprocessing or EMDR, talk therapy (including for moral injuries), and magnet therapy. In addition, many veterans with PTSD struggle with alcohol or drug use, and Vet Center provides treatment for substance abuse.

3. A private counselor might be able to help someone with PTSD with a variety of techniques. Although these are not paid for by the VA, they may help someone for whom the other therapies previously mentioned have not been effective. These treatments include: brief eclectic psychotherapy (BEC), narrative exposure therapy (NET), or cognitive behavioral therapy (CBT). Some therapists may choose to work specifically on the symptoms of PTSD, with therapies like stress inoculation training (SIT), present-centered therapy (PCT), or interpersonal psychotherapy (IPT).

4. There are a variety of churches and ministries that provide free counseling or low-cost counseling to veterans and others affected by PTSD. One organization that my family personally had a positive experience with was the Welcome Home Initiative, which offers weekend conferences for veterans and their spouses free of charge. They combine prayer with more traditional counseling.

5. There are a variety of organizations that train dogs as service animals for veterans with PTSD. These animals can be trained to wake a person during a nightmare, to help someone sit down and take slow breaths when their heart rate is elevated. They can perform a variety of other functions. A lot of these

organizations are regional, since the veteran and the dog both have to be trained together for a period of time.

6. Some people have found help through complementary therapies, including: yoga, acupuncture, essential oil therapy, mindfulness meditation, homeopathy, herbal therapy, or regular visits to a chiropractor.

7. New treatments are coming out each year. James Rosone has found great success with stellate ganglion nerve blocks (which help reset the physical fight or flight symptoms of PTSD) and ketamine therapy (which helps to reset the brain itself).

The purpose of this section is not to tell you what therapy may be right for you or your loved one, but to give you HOPE and a starting place when seeking out help. For sake of space, I did not define all the terms here, but please feel free to check them all out. Sometimes it may take time before the right treatment is found. Please do not give up!

If you feel like you are stuck and need someone to reach out to, please feel free to email me, Miranda Watson, or my husband, James Rosone, at james.rosone@gmail.com, and we will do our best to help you move on to the next step. No man or woman left behind.

Made in United States
North Haven, CT
02 December 2023